Jeff KISSI

Women and the ethics of procreation

Jeff KISSI

Women and the ethics of procreation

Virginity-Menstruation - Desirable births

ScienciaScripts

Imprint
Any brand names and product names mentioned in this book are subject to trademark, brand or patent protection and are trademarks or registered trademarks of their respective holders. The use of brand names, product names, common names, trade names, product descriptions etc. even without a particular marking in this work is in no way to be construed to mean that such names may be regarded as unrestricted in respect of trademark and brand protection legislation and could thus be used by anyone.

Cover image: www.ingimage.com

This book is a translation from the original published under ISBN 978-620-6-70515-4.

Publisher:
Sciencia Scripts
is a trademark of
Dodo Books Indian Ocean Ltd. and OmniScriptum S.R.L publishing group

120 High Road, East Finchley, London, N2 9ED, United Kingdom
Str. Armeneasca 28/1, office 1, Chisinau MD-2012, Republic of Moldova, Europe
Printed at: see last page
ISBN: 978-620-7-71844-3

Contents

Preface

by Professor Emerite Stanis Wembonyama

DËDICACE

To Jesus Christ, the all-knowing one, we are grateful for the wisdom and intelligence we have received, and we do so graciously!

To my dearly beloved mother Lydie MASUDI, not only for your constant efforts to ensure my education, but also for giving me a taste for study and for your tolerance of my whims from birth to the present day.

To all of you, from far and near, who contributed to the writing of this book: les couples Professeur Emerite Stanis WEMBONYAMA, BEEN MASUDI, Mister BEEN MASUDI, Christian MBUYU, Me Felix KANDOLO, Me Tom MOMA, Steve BEEN MASUDI, John MBUYI, Michel KAPEND, MASANGU MBOMBO, les Pasteurs Emmanuel MULONGO, Sylvano KAPAYA, Don Samuel LANDU, Benjamin AHOKA, Nicky KANDJA, Romain MANDE, Pierrot MUKANYA, Dr. Dr. Cheikh BICIMU, Dr. Christian TSHIMTSHIOMPO, Dr. Philippe MULENGA, Dr. Emery IBEKI, Dr. Celia BICIMU Emery IBEKI, Dr Celestin PONGOMBO, as well as the brothers and sisters Deborah ILUNGA, Gaël NDALA, Toussaint MAYOMBO, Shadrack TSHITALA, the twins Shadrack and Meschack BWANGA, Josaphat KATOMBYO, Josias KAYUMBA, Syntiche KABWE, Joël fiston ILUNGA, Patrick-fortune KASONGO, Milord MUTONDO, Marc KABENGELE, Jogi Jean-Luc IRUNG, Paul TSHIPENG, Timothee KABWE, Gracia KIFUAME, Ines MWAMBA, Giody Audrey KANYINDA, all the members of Espace Kyubo, all the companions of Public Health, for your advice and support during the conception and writing of this book.

We would also like to thank all those who agreed to take part in the survey.

I would like to thank all those whose names have not been mentioned for their spiritual, moral and material support.

Jeff KISSI K.

PREFACE

This book, which Mr Jeff Kissi has done us the honour of prefacing, is at the heart of morality and the stability of couples and families. This book confronts us with our responsibilities in terms of the choices we have to make to ensure the well-being of our unborn children and that of our societies.

The intellectual output of Mr Jeff Kissi, the author of this book, takes us on a journey into ethical and religious values, and raises questions about how we all see our society today, in terms of the confrontation between good and evil, between charitable practices and the trivialisation of existential problems likely to shock purists.

These actions are likely to label the protagonists as people working to reduce the population, which is contrary to the religion, which is pronatalist. However, in this book, there is no question of limiting births by preventing women from procreating.

The issues addressed in this book are based on practices that are already being carried out illegally in some countries, with glaring failures due to ignorance, the greed of certain health bodies and the absence of proper laws on thorny and topical social issues. Failure to address these issues means opening the door to unwanted pregnancies, with their cortege of criminal abortions, harmful consequences for women's health, repercussions on the balance within families, and the stigmatisation and criminalisation of certain practices.

Whether we are talking about menstruation, contraception or virginity, Jeff Kissi's book clearly sets out the role of education, the implications for health, behaviour within the family, making couples more responsible and, by extension, methods for avoiding side-effects, health problems and harmful economic consequences.

We can only congratulate the author for drawing on his extensive knowledge and expertise and his position as a man of God, one who sounds the alarm to prevent and preserve our society from the horrors caused by harmful practices.

Finally, we appeal to churchmen, temporal powers, parents, young people and legislators to draw inspiration from the realities described in this book, which is both fascinating to read and to write. This is how we will be able to advise, guide and support young people, adults and parents in their efforts to ensure their well-being on the earth of the living.

Professor WEMBONYAMA OKITOTSHO Stanis

Professor Emeritus of Paediatrics and Public Health, Full Member of the Academy of Sciences,

Writer, poet, philosopher, journalist, honorary national deputy, state dignitary,

Medaille d'or de merite civique, Medaille d'or des arts, sciences et lettres,

Diplome de merite scientifique et academique, Diplome du serment d'Hippocrate de l'ordre des medecins
Honorary diploma from Congolese universities,
Honorary Rector of the Universities, Dean of the Faculties of Medicine,
Physician at the University Clinics of the University of Lubumbashi.

INTRODUCTION

The book, which we have the humility to present to the public, has been produced to help young working people acquire knowledge on a range of subjects on which they are not only ill-informed and/or under-informed, but also exposed to the taboos that underpin and dictate behaviour in our society.
These young people are influenced by intox* and/or infox* in terms of the information they glean here and there, which has led them to the deplorable disinformation and disorientation that have taken on worrying proportions.
Young people are a major force and a source of hope for the future of an entire nation and even for the next generation, and they are entitled to a coherent basic education and training. The difficulties we encountered during our interviews with some young people on a variety of subjects, including human reproduction, family planning, virginity, menstruation, marriage, betrothal, celibacy, etc. - the list is not exhaustive - reinforce our conviction that we should make this knowledge available to them.
So the problem of human reproduction remains a subject of interest to all generations, and one that deserves our full attention in this book, entitled "***Women and the Ethics of Procreation".***
This book is the culmination of our combined efforts in reading, researching different taboo subjects, our personal experience and re-evaluating the level of knowledge among young people of both sexes.
The Maputo Protocol, adopted in 2003, is one of the first legal frameworks for the protection of the **rights** and freedoms of women and young girls in **Africa**. It recognises access to medical **abortion** under certain conditions as a human **right** that women should enjoy without restriction, even though the Penal Code continues to punish those who induce abortion and women who voluntarily agree to abort[1 2] .
Article 14 of the Maputo Protocol is the only legal instrument dealing with the right of women and girls in Africa to have access to safe abortion. This provision guarantees ***"the reproductive rights of women, in particular by authorising medical abortion in cases of sexual assault, rape, incest and when the pregnancy endangers the mental and physical health of the mother or the***

** Intox is the diminutive of "intoxication", which comes from the verb intoxicate and means insidious action on the mind to confirm an opinion, demoralise, influence... **Infox** is also considered to be fake news, false information, misleading information, canards, in English: fake news, is untruthful news disseminated with the aim of manipulating or deceiving the public.

[2] Art. 165 and 166 of the Congolese Criminal Code.

life of the mother or the foetus"[3] .

Although most countries in sub-Saharan Africa have ratified the Maputo Protocol, only seven[4] have undertaken legal reform to harmonise their laws and incorporate the Protocol's provisions on access to safe abortion.

Meanwhile, the news in 2022 warns that in the United States, all eyes are on the Supreme Court. The institution has been at the heart of a virulent political, legal and social debate since the publication, on Monday 2 May by the *Politico* website, of a draft ruling by America's highest judicial body that could overturn the famous Roe v. Wade case law of 1973, which protects the right of American women to terminate their pregnancies. If adopted as it stands, this ruling would set the United States back fifty years, to a time when each state was free to authorise voluntary termination of pregnancy (abortion) or to ban it[5] .

This book is also the fruit of our experience in higher education and university, where we have accumulated a certain amount of knowledge not only in this particular field, but also in many other areas of life, which has enabled us to develop and broaden our knowledge. It has been written to guide young people in their work, and why not adults who are also concerned by the same problem.

This book "***La Femme et I'Ethique de la procreation***" is based on a survey carried out among young girls and boys from the Gecamines district in the Commune of Lubumbashi and those from the Cadastre district in the Commune of Kampemba, as well as some married couples, all from the city of Lubumbashi. These are the victims of intoxication in the life issues addressed throughout this book, the writing of which began in May 2018.

This book is intended as a modest contribution to the edification of youth and posterity, in the hope that it will undoubtedly serve as a benchmark for further research by others in the same field. The research was vital, as it enabled us to provide a detailed response to the above-mentioned problem.

We would like to take this opportunity to thank Professor Emeritus Dr Stanis WEMBONYAMA for his availability and constant advice, as it was his many scientific publications that sharpened our own flair and inspired the writing of this book.

[3] African Commission on Human and Peoples' Rights, Protocol to the African Charter on Human and Peoples' Rights on the Rights of Women in Africa

[4] eSwatini, Eritrea, Mauritius, Mozambique, the Democratic Republic of Congo, Rwanda and Chad. Two countries, Sao Tome and Principe and Benin (as of October 2021), have exceeded the Maputo Protocol.

[5] *Avortement aux Etats-Unis : un retour en arriere de la Cour supreme serait " l'aboutissement" de cinquante ans de " combat de la droite religieuse contre l'IVG "* in **Journal Le Monde** edition du 7 mai 2022.

CHAPTER I

VIRGINITY

What is virginity?

The question of virginity is often linked to that of the hymen, the thin, flexible membrane at the entrance to the vagina.
Virginity means never having had sexual relations. The woman or young girl is then described as a "virgin". It is during the first sexual intercourse, whether voluntary or forced, that the young girl/woman loses her virginity[6] .

Is virginity physical or moral?

Virginity is a concept that refers to the state of never having had sexual relations. Virginity has no biological basis, but is a social, cultural and religious fact. What is at stake is the virginity of women (*especially* unmarried women), while that of men is of little importance. It is often associated with notions of purity and honour, particularly in cultures and religions that insist on abstinence before marriage[7] .
The cultural and social importance of virginity has necessitated a number of different techniques for verifying the virginity of a future bride. First and foremost, the hymen is supposed to break during vaginal penetration. In some cultures and periods, virginity tests or the presence of blood on the sheets after the wedding night were used to prove the virtue of the bride, although they were not reliable indicators: the first sexual encounter with penetration did not systematically cause the hymen to break. Virginity is impossible to establish medically.
Commonly, when we talk about virginity, everyone refers to sex (deflowering of the hymen).
Done :
Mrs NGOY is a virgin, she says, because she has never had or had sexual intercourse with a man. However, she practices **fellatio (a** sexual practice that consists of sucking, licking and inserting her partner's sex into her mouth**), sodomy** (penetration through the anus) **and masturbation. When she is married, will she still be considered a virgin?** It's up to you, the reader, to answer.
For this reason, the question of virginity should not necessarily be based on sexual contact of the vaginal orifice with a being of the opposite sex, but rather

[6] Le Dictionnaire de l'Academie frangaise, "Deflorer" [archive], Centre national de ressources textuelles et lexicales (sens 2) [consulted 19 November 2016].
[7] Ditto

on any act that compromises the modesty of the female being.
The female being of the 21eme century having the knowledge of virginity as being a phenomenon that is measured by sexual contact, has developed so many erotic practices to circumvent the pleasure of the sexual act by defying the above definition of virginity, to say that she has never had sexual intercourse, thus saying that she is a complete virgin.
If today we continue to define virginity by the simple fact of sexual intercourse through intromission into the female sexual organ, it means that we are wrong. Virginity, in this day and age, is a sacred word that cannot be used to describe a pure, healthy, integrated person, and **only God can best measure virginity by means of his indicators, we believe**.
Hence, the true measure **of virginity lies in the conscience of each being.** For conscience is the only element that no one can ever defy or deceive, no matter what acts or schemes are carried out in secret to deceive human vigilance.
Let's take another taboo word that is also the subject of intoxication in this century: **"*hymen*".**

What is the hymen?

The **hymen** (from йиф' / *hym&n*, meaning:
The "membrane" is a membrane which, in women and several mammal species, partially closes the opening of the vagina and separates the vaginal cavity from the vulva.
It is important to stress that not all women have a hymen, and contrary to popular belief, when it is present, it does not necessarily tear during the first sexual intercourse with vaginal penetration, but relaxes[8] .

Embryological origin

The hymen is derived from the interface between the urogenital sinus and the Mullerian ducts, which opened into each other to form the uterus. On contact with the urogenital sinus (vaginal orifice), the mesodermal ***"Mullerian"*** tissue thickens and then vacuolates. The vacuole will open on the side of the urogenital sinus and form the hymen, but also on the side of the ***Mullerian*** ducts, which will form the cervix.

Role of the hymen

"The hymen has no specific role. We can say that in little girls, it protects the inside of the vagina to some extent, but it has neither a physiological nor a sexological role. The only use for the hymen would perhaps be cultural and religious as a symbol of virginity, but it remains only a symbol".

[8] Biology course, 6e des humanites Scientifiques, Cs des eloges, 2013

Is the hymen firm

Many women and men have told us that the hymen is something that is hermetically sealed, however, ***by definition it is open*** *as it allows the menstruation to pass through. It's important to point out that this ring is elastic, which means that even at first intercourse, it won't necessarily tear, it will just stretch. What's more, bleeding on first intercourse is not compulsory. You should know that more than* ***half of women do not bleed.*** *You can be a literal virgin and not bleed at first intercourse*[9] *.*

Types or forms of hymen

There are several forms of the hymen and these forms vary from one woman to another, depending on her morphology:

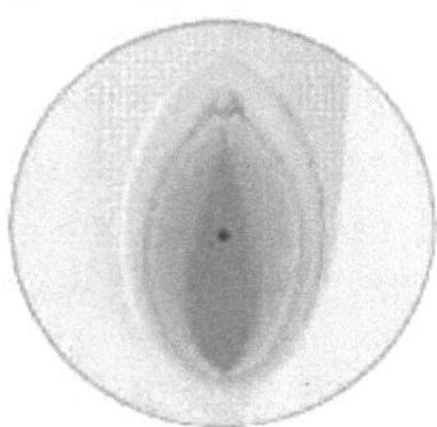

- **Imperforate hymen**: membrane covering the entrance to the vagina. In this case, the menstrual periods cannot flow. In this case, the hymen needs to be incised to perforate it.

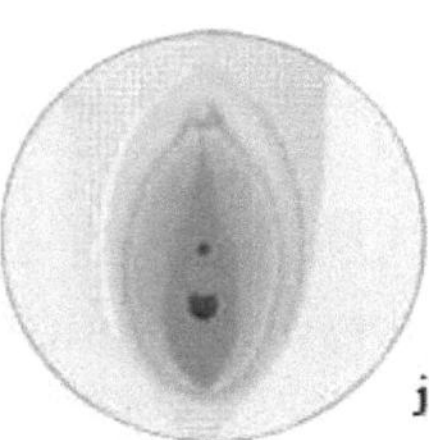

- **Microperforated hymen**: the membrane covers almost the entire entrance to the vagina, the perforation of the hymen being very small.

- In general, the rules are flowing but the

young girls will not be able to insert or remove a tampon because the hymen is too small. In this case, a small incision in the hymen is needed to enlarge the opening.

[9] Ditto

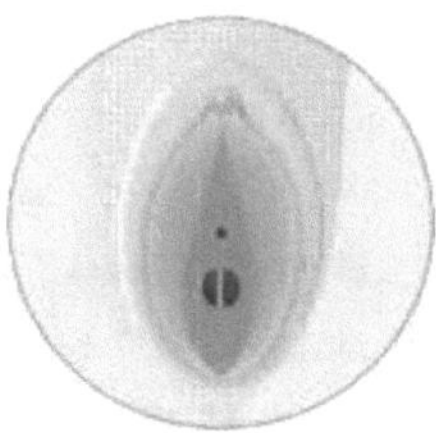

- **Hymen *bifenetre***: the membrane has two small openings in the vagina instead of one. All that's needed is a minor operation to remove a small strip of tissue to create a normal opening.

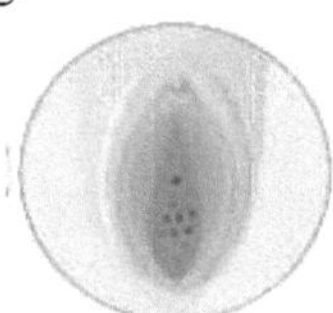

- ***Cribriform* hymen**: membrane with multiple small holes.
- ***Sclerotic* hymen**: thick, tough membrane that makes sexual relations difficult.

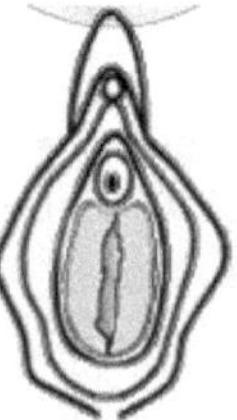

Complacent hymen: elastic membrane that dilates without bleeding or tearing.

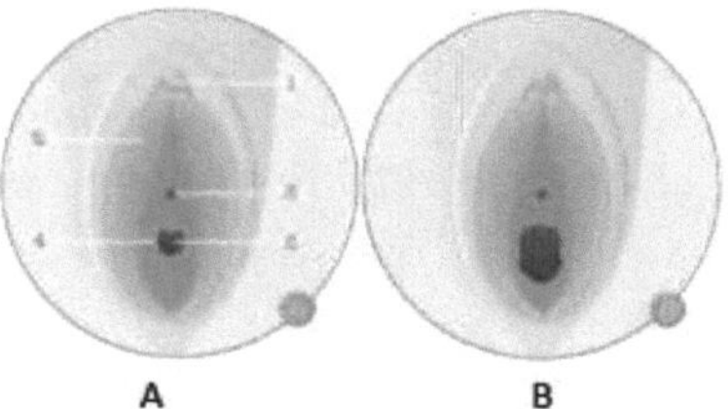

1. Clitoris / 2. Small lips / 3. Urinary meatus / 4. Hymen / 5. vaginal orifice

A: Hymen intact B: Hymen dechire

Do I bleed when I first have vaginal intercourse?

Contrary to widespread belief, bleeding does not necessarily occur at first intercourse. Bleeding is not automatic, and some women lose a few drops of blood when the hymen tears. This tear can sometimes be painful, but it can also go unnoticed.

Some hymens are more vascular than others, causing bleeding when they rupture. Conversely, others do not bleed at first intercourse. Almost 50% of women do not bleed at first intercourse[10] .

Is the hymen an indicator of virginity?

We have received several testimonies and been informed of several cases of divorce following the question of the hymen (tearing of the hymen accompanied by bleeding) which many men use to determine the virginity of their spouses at the time of the wedding, and if at the time of the first sexual intercourse with vaginal penetration the man does not see the presence of blood, he immediately believes that the woman is unfaithful and claims to be the victim of a lie.

Fact:

Mrs **NVITA** had never known any men in her life until she was married to Mr **KITWA**. On the wedding night, he discovered that his wife had a ruptured hymen because she had not bled during intercourse or when the penis was inserted into the vagina. The man had not felt any resistance or difficulty in penetrating. However, Mrs NVITA had sworn to her husband before the wedding that she had never known any man apart from her husband (KITWA), and this on the wedding night.

Mr KITWA was furious and no longer wanted to listen to his wife, so he decided to divorce her immediately after the wedding. But before the divorce was finalized, Mr KITWA met his former classmate, Mr **NDALA**. Mr Ndala was not only his friend, but also a member of the medical profession. KITWA began to recount his wedding misadventure. When he had finished, Mr Ndala smiled calmly and asked Mr Kitta if he really trusted his wife. Mr KITWA agreed, even saying that he loved his wife very much. Mr Ndala took the opportunity to dispel the ideas put forward by his friend Kittawa on the question of virginity linked to bleeding during first intercourse by telling him the following:

The definition of virginity varies according to time and culture. It can be understood as the absence of any sexual intercourse, or it can be limited to the absence of vaginal penetration. The presence of fhymen as a criterion of virginity means that a girl who has had sodomy, rubbing or fellatio but whose hymen is intact is considered a virgin, whereas a girl who has not had sexual intercourse with anyone but practices masturbation would be considered a non-virgin if she has broken her hymen.

However, the definitions of sexual intercourse can vary enough that many acts

[10] "Au Maroc, la virginite a tout prix : " Ils veulent du sang, alors on leur en donne " ", Journal Le Monde, 24 September 2017 (read online [archive], consulted on 7 January 2020).

are either included or excluded. A survey of teenagers shows that 2% consider themselves to be non-virgins after a deep kiss, 15% if they touch someone else's genitals or vice versa, 40% if they are involved in an act of oral sex, 99.5% after a coi't (the questions are of the yes/no type)[11] .

Those who point to kissing as a loss of virginity may also point to others. For American teenagers, sex without penetration is a way of remaining a "technical virgin". These definitions are themselves the subject of debate in the United States, where the Christian vision of virginity implies the absence of any sexual act whatsoever[12] .

Similarly, voluntariness is taken into account in the concept of virginity: in some cultures, rape does not result in the loss of virginity because the woman did not consent. Saint Augustine specifies that consent is necessary to lose virginity. In other words, rape does not remove virginity[13] .

In many cultures around the world, the loss of a woman's virginity must take place on the wedding night. A virginity examination may be carried out before the wedding (through an inspection of the hymen). The blood-stained sheet may be displayed after the wedding night to prove that the woman has arrived at the wedding as a virgin and that the first sexual intercourse has just taken place. This is the case in North Africa, Vietnam and Armenia (the ceremony is called the "red apple").

In Tonga, bloodstained sheets are inspected by the bride's family and then handed over to the groom's family[14] .

In other African countries (Haut-Katanga, Lualaba, Maniema, etc. in the DRC), the bride and groom have sex on a white cloth while their families wait. As soon as the intercourse is over, the women from the groom's family check the cloth for blood. The bride's family, overjoyed, then present the cloth to the other members of the family, showing that their daughter was indeed a virgin.

Other eyewitness accounts point to complicity between the two spouses, who had known each other before, and who managed to injure each other in order to stain or smear blood on the sheets and show that it had been a deflowering.

Conversely, if there is no bloodshed, an investigation is carried out by both families and if it concludes that the wife is not a virgin, the husband may repudiate her in order to mitigate the dishonour felt. The woman's family can also dishonour her. In Wallis, a special area is set aside for the bride and groom in the bride's house; the day after the wedding night, the bridegroom brings the

[11] "La virginite, qu'est-ce que c'est?" [archive], on Fil sante jeunes (consulted on 7 January 2020).

[12] Journal des femmes, Paris

[13] Journal des femmes, Op.cit paris

[14] Trong Hieu Dinh, "Vraies et fausses vierges au Viet Nam. La falsification corporelle en question", Extreme-Orient Extreme-Occident, n° 32, 1[er] October 2010, p. 163-191.

blood-stained sheet and is escorted home by his family, who bring gifts. Similarly, in some cultures in the DRC, the gift is in kind: goats, chickens or cows.

However, some women are born without a hymen. Furthermore, the hymen can break without penetration, during the practice of a sport such as *Kange*, classical dance, karate, jumping, horse riding, motorcycling, cycling or during childhood growth without the woman realising. On the other hand, some women can be penetrated by a penis without the hymen even being relaxed (*complaisant hymen*) and the hymen will only break during childbirth.

"The hymen is an unreliable element in determining the virginity of a woman or a girl. The presence or absence of a hymen can only be determined by visual examination by an experienced (zil).

But if the hymen is torn or perforated, this does not prove that the woman is no longer a virgin (common parlance). If the hymen is intact, this does not prove anything either, as it can be elastic and allow itself to be penetrated without breaking. The only thing that can be established with medical certainty is the absence of the hymen, not the way in which it has disappeared. Once the hymen has been removed, it cannot be regenerated.

Therefore, dear men, beware of this habit (legend) of seeing blood on the white sheet to prove your wife's virginity. Certain stratagems are put in place to ensure that the sheets are indeed bloodstained, as indicated above.

For example, a cock can be killed and its blood used instead of the woman's. Since the 2000s, artificial hymen and hymenoplasty have also been used.

Certain surgical procedures can be used to reconstruct the hymen or give the impression that it is intact, such as hymenoplasty.

In Germany, as in France, several *"hymenkliniken"* (people who perform hymen surgery) specialise in hymen reconstruction surgery.

There are two types of surgery. One involves sewing up the torn hymen membrane with a very fine thread one or two days before the wedding. The other can be carried out up to two weeks before the wedding and is performed with slow resorption sutures. In West Africa, midwives are renowned for performing this type of operation, with all the risks of infection.

Each of these operations is quick and benign, and requires only a little local anaesthetic. However, hymen reconstruction does not guarantee bleeding during vaginal penetration.

There are also artificial hymens, the purpose of which is to simulate the loss of blood that sometimes follows first intercourse. This consists of a small translucent artificial pouch containing a red liquid made up of natural albumin, which the woman places in her vagina around twenty minutes before intercourse. Under the effect of body heat, the membrane dilates, creating a sensation of deflation during penetration. The red liquid spreads and stains the sheets with a few drops, simulating the rupture of the hymen. This 'virginity kit' was invented in Japan in the 1990s and is now used worldwide[15] .

To conclude this subject, and to give a definitive answer to Mr KITWA, who initiated the divorce process because his wife did not bleed on the wedding night, and for all the reasons given above***, the hymen cannot be considered as a guarantee of a woman's virginity, any less than bleeding on the wedding night.***

Finally, Mr KITWA, now informed, has rescinded his divorce decision and he and his wife are living happily together today.

You too, who are reading this book, may be in the same situation as Mr KITWA and Mrs NVITA, his wife, or you may know someone who is in a similar situation. Please share what you have gained from reading this book. Save a couple! And let's all block the road to marital intoxication.

♦♦

[15] Journal des femmes, Op.cit. paris

CHAPTER II

MENSTRUATION

What is menstruation (Les regies)

The term *menstruation* comes from the Latin word *mensis,* meaning "month" (closely related to the Greek *mene,* the moon), which suggests a connection with the monthly lunar cycles.

By definition, periods are **the flow of blood that occurs once a month in a woman**. They are scientifically referred to as menstruation, because they are part of the menstrual cycle, which prepares the body for a possible pregnancy[16] . Menstruation is also referred to as menstruation, which means the monthly flow of blood in non-pregnant people[17] .

Menstruation, or **periods,** refers to the periodic flow of a complex biological fluid made up of blood, vaginal secretions and endometrial cells from the uterine wall, discharged through the vagina[18] .

Where does the blood come from?

The origin of the blood in the uterus is explained in medicine. The regia correspond to the elimination of a membrane lining the uterus called the endometrium.

- Each month, the **endometrium thickens** under the effect of astrogen, a female hormone, to form a nest ready to receive an embryo.
- In the middle of the cycle, **one of the ovaries releases a** mature **egg**: this is called ovu l ation.
- If the egg is not fertilised by a spermatozoon, the ovum dies within 24 to 72 hours, and **the endometrium breaks down and is eliminated by the body**. This is where the blood in the uterus comes from.

Premenstrual syndrome (Early signs)

The term premenstrual syndrome covers **a series of symptoms** that many women experience **a few days before their period**. They can sometimes be a little unpleasant, but they let you know that your period is about to start. Here are the most common:

- Temporary weight gain of 1 or 2 kg ;
- Enervated, irritable;
- Slight depression ;
- Bloating or abdominal cramps ;

[16] Cours de Biologie, op.cit.
[17] Larousse French dictionary.
[18] Ditto

- Tension in the breasts ;
- Headaches;
- Acne growth.

For some women, menstruation triggers migraines. This is a very specific type of migraine that heralds the arrival of menstruation, known as catamenial migraines. Menstruation can also cause constipation, or conversely temporary diarrhoea[19] .

What is the normal duration of menstruation?

The duration of menstruation varies greatly from one woman to another and from one age to another. On average, it lasts from **2 to 7 days**, with a heavier flow during the first two days.

How can I calculate the date of my next period?

Menstruation occurs 14 days after the day of ovulation, which is often difficult to know in advance. To calculate the date of your period, you need to know how many days your menstrual cycle lasts.

- By definition, a cycle begins on the first day of menstruation and ends on the last day before the next menstruation.
- We often talk about 28-day cycles, but the average length is between 28 and 33 days.
- Some women even have cycles that are significantly **shorter** (21 days) or **longer** (up to 35 days), which is completely normal.

Are my regies normal?

It's a question that some women often ask themselves when faced with heavy or very light periods. But even if they seem heavy, they lose a maximum of 80 ml of blood, the average being around 45 ml. If the discharge is excessive, it may be menorrhagia (heavy vaginal bleeding)[20] or haemorrhagic periods.

Irregular rules

Weak periods are normal in young girls at the start of puberty. It can also happen that periods start earlier than expected: irregular cycles are normal in young girls.

[19] Cours de Biologie, op.cit.
[20] Cours de biologie, op.cit.

Black registers

Darker or lighter periods are not necessarily a sign of a gynaecological problem. However, if your mucous membranes are smelly or you have an unusual, thick, foul-smelling discharge, you could be suffering from vaginosis (an increase in the number of microbes [bacteria] in the vagina). This is usually due to an imbalance in the vaginal flora (acid or microbes that protect the vagina from other microbes).

Painful periods

To eliminate the endometrial mucosa, the muscles of the uterus must contract. This can cause sometimes severe pain in the abdomen at the time of menstruation. These periods are called **dysmenorrhoea**. If the pain is very frequent or recurs during sexual intercourse, it may be due to a condition known as endometriosis, which affects around 10% of women[20] .

The pains are often more **intense in the first few years in young girls**; there is nothing systematic about them. Some women feel nothing at all, while others simply feel a slight tension in their lower abdomen. If your periods become really difficult to bear, a doctor or midwife will be able to offer you a solution and check that there is no particular pathology.

However, you should always beware of grandmother's recipes, which suggest the same medicine based on leaf or root tea for any pain in the lower abdomen, without knowing the dose. This medication is the cause of sterility in some women. It is therefore advisable to consult a specialist before taking any kind of medicine or herbal tea.

The absence of registers

Are you experiencing a delay in your cycle? There are several explanations for the temporary absence or delay of your period:

1. Some women have **irregular periods all their lives**, it's in their nature.
2. But many other women can have cycles that 'skip' a month or two depending on **life's events**. Travelling, **major stress**, illness or a change in diet can all lead to a temporary absence of periods.
3. If this is not the case, **pregnancy is** obviously **a possibility**, especially if you have had sexual intercourse without contraception.
4. Finally, during the menopause, the reproductive cycle stops: there are no more periods.

Menstrual periods in pregnant women

Bleeding that resembles menstruation may occur in the first few months of pregnancy. This is generally minor bleeding that corresponds to the implantation of the gestational sac in the uterus or to the first changes in the body.

There's another phenomenon: anniversary bleeding (bleeding that occurs on the day you should have your next period but while you're pregnant). A bleed occurs on the date when you should be having your period while you are pregnant. **It's not a real menstruation,** but it's obviously quite unnerving. A doctor or midwife will be able to reassure you in this rare case[21] .

Phases of the menstrual cycle

The first is called the follicular phase

During this period, more and more hormones - called astrogens - are produced. They cause the uterine mucosa to thicken and the number of blood vessels to increase.

The second phase

During this time, an egg in one of the ovaries has matured and is expelled. This **is the phase known as ovulation**. The egg travels down the fallopian tube towards the uterus, which is now ready to receive it. At this point, the amount of oestrogen in the woman's body begins to decrease.

The third phase, known as the progestational (or luteal) phase, begins.

It is characterised by the development of a corpus luteum which secretes another hormone, progesterone. Progesterone is also responsible for preparing the uterus for implantation of the egg, if the ovum has been fertilised by a sperm. To do this, the uterus is filled with blood, tissue, sugar, protein, etc.

The fourth phase

If the egg has not been fertilised in the days following its passage through the fallopian tube, progesterone levels also begin to fall. **The unfertilised egg eventually dissolves and the excess uterine wall detaches**. The whole thing is then evacuated as "blood" to the outside, via the cervix and vagina. This **is the fourth phase: the period or menstrual phase**.

What is the period when the regia are located in relation to the time when the ovum can be fertilised?

The first day of a woman's cycle is the first day of her period. The last day is the day before the next period. Whatever the number of days between two periods, menstruation always occurs fourteen days after ovulation. However, the length of time before ovulation varies.

Calculating the date of ovulation: short or long cycle.

Two couples in ten (10) find it difficult to space their children because they are unfamiliar with the best time to have fertile sexual relations. Six out of ten (6

[21] Sexual health, Paris 2020

out of 10) adolescents have unwanted pregnancies because they do not know how to calculate their ovulatory period[22 23] .

The **female cycle** begins **on the first day of menstruation** and ends on the first day of the next period. So, if the first day of menstruation is the 3[e] day of the month and the 1[er] day of the next menstrual period is the 31[eme] day of the month, the **cyclewill last28 days**.

The menstrual cycle is made up of **4 phases**:

- **The follicular phase** (around 14 days, including 5 days of menstruation),
- **Ovulation** (24 or 72 hours on average)
- **The luteal phase** (around 14 days)
- **The menstrual phase** (around 5 to 7 days of menstruation).

Diagram of the female cycle[23]

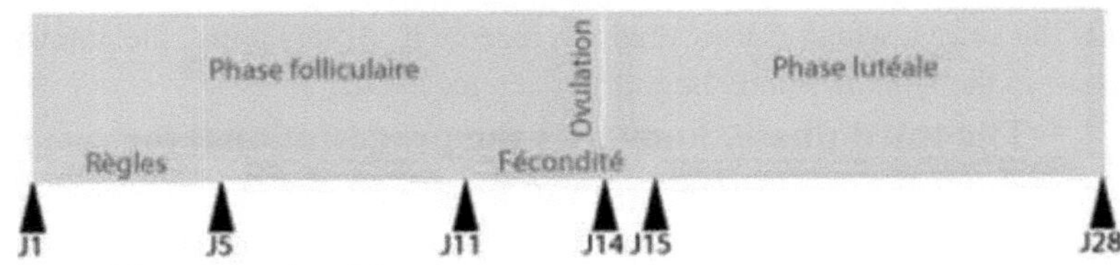

(Diagram of the menstrual cycle)

What is ovulation?

Ovulation is the expulsion of the oocyte (egg) from the ovary, ready to be fertilised by a spermatozoon and give birth to an embryo. Ovulation is a continuous physiological process that begins at puberty and ends at the menopause. At the menopause, the activity of the ovaries ceases and the woman no longer ovulates or has regia.

As long as the menopause has not fully set in, she (the woman) is still ovulating and pregnancy is still possible.

Lifespan of the egg and spermatozoa

The egg lives for around **12 to 72 hours** after being expelled from the ovary. The spermatozoa survive in the cervix and remain fecund for around **3 to 5 days**.

22 Sante sexuelle, op.cit.

23 Journal des Femmes Sante

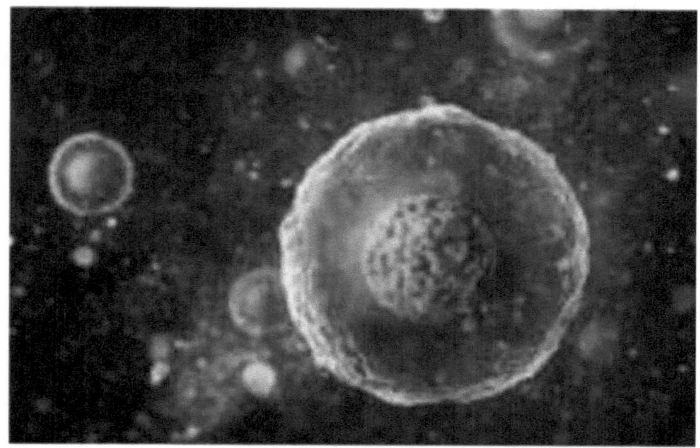

What is an ovum?

The egg cell is a female reproductive cell up to three times larger than the sperm cell. Between puberty and the menopause, a woman will produce between **300** and **400** of them, at a rate of one egg every month (sometimes two)[24] .

Symptoms(Signs) of the ovulation period

The ovulation period can manifest itself through a whole range of more or less marked symptoms, such as :

- Sensation of breast tension,
- Abdominal pain occurring on the side of the ovary which releases its oocyte,
- Presence for 2 or 3 days of cervical mucus (mucus which protects the vagina from infection) and transparent, slightly sticky vaginal secretions with a consistency similar to egg white,
- Sensation of increased libido.

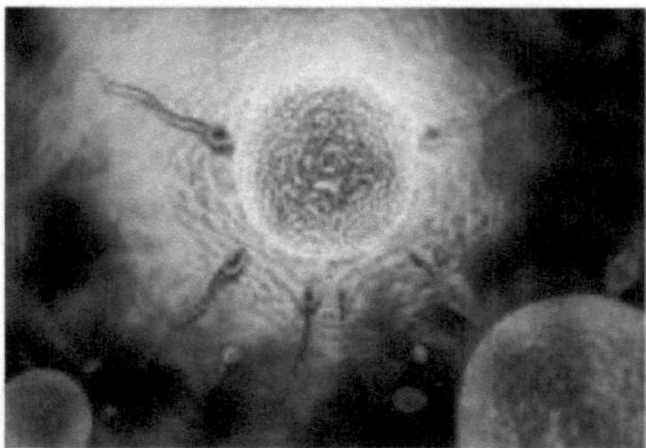

The absence of these symptoms does not mean that there has been no ovulation Ovulation generally occurs two weeks before the onset of menstruation in women with regular cycles. For women with irregular cycles, it can be useful to look out for the signs of ovulation, particularly if you want to get pregnant.

Post-ovulatory phase

The post-ovulatory phase lasts **14 days** in theory for a regular 28-day cycle, but can last from **10 to 20 days** in the case of very irregular cycles.

THE FECONDATION

Fertilisation is a fundamental stage in sexual reproduction, during which the male gamete fuses with the female gamete to form the egg, known as the **zygote**.

In humans, the spermatozoon is the male gamete and the egg is the female gamete. The sperm contained in the semen emitted into the woman's vaginal cavity will come into contact with the egg, and one of them will penetrate the egg. After penetration, the oocyte will become "hermetically sealed" to the entry of other spermatozoa, allowing **a single egg** to **develop**[25] .

Fertilisation therefore corresponds to the fusion phase between an ovum and a spermatozoon, resulting in a single cell that will become the embryo. If fertilisation does not occur, there is a sudden drop in hormone levels and the onset of menstruation. If fertilisation occurs, a specific pregnancy hormone is produced: **HCG** *(human chorionic gonadotropin: hormone produced by the placenta*). This hormone helps to maintain the production of other hormones and therefore to keep the endometrium intact so that the future embryo can "settle" there[26] .

The best time to conceive a baby, known as the **fertile period**, is between the day before and just after the ovulation phase, i.e. between the fourth day before ovulation and 24 hours after. Four days before and one day after the fourteenth day of the cycle are favourable days for fertilisation in a 28-day cycle, i.e. in a normal cycle, between the tenth and fifteenth day of the cycle. When fertilisation cannot take place naturally, in vitro fertilisation can be used, which involves the formation of an egg outside the woman's body, which is then transferred to her uterus. This operation or method is expensive and may be recommended to couples who are having difficulty.

Fertile period: how to calculate it, difference with ovulation

A woman's fertility is cyclical. The fertile period is the phase of the menstrual cycle during which a woman can conceive. How is it calculated? What is the difference with ovulation? Is it possible to become pregnant outside the fecundity period?

Fertilisation if you have a normal cycle:

► Date of ovulation

A normal cycle lasts 28 days. Ovulation occurs on day 14[eme] . This ovulation

[25] Cours de biologie, op. cit.
[26] Journal des femmes, Op.cit

date is used to determine the fertility period. Ovulation, which lasts 24 hours, corresponds to the release of the oocyte by the ovary. The 14eme day of the menstrual cycle, out of a regular 28-day cycle, remains **the most fertile period**. The first day of the cycle is the first day of menstruation. It should be noted that just because ovulation occurs halfway through a regular cycle (28 days) does not mean that it always occurs halfway through the cycle (for example, on day 16eme of a 32-day cycle, or day 12eme of a 24-day cycle). The egg is generally expelled **14 days** before the start of your period. So, if you have irregular cycles and cannot anticipate the date of your next period, it will be more difficult to determine the date of ovulation. The use of a temperature curve or ovulation tests can be considered.

► Fertility period

The best fertile period is before and just after the ovulation phase, i.e. from around 4eme days before ovulation to 24 hours afterwards. **4 days before and 1 day after the fourteenth day** of the ovulation cycle are days that are favourable for fertilisation in a 28-day cycle, i.e. in the case of a normal cycle, between the 10th^{eme} day and the 15th^{eme} day of the cycle. If the length of the menstrual cycle is longer than 35 days, shorter than 21 days, or if the menstrual cycle tends to be irregular, the results of this calculation may not be exactly the same[27] .

Fertile days

We'll illustrate this calculation with a concrete example of Mrs NGOY, who has a regular, normal 28-day cycle; the periodicity or frequency of her periods is 3 days.

Example: Mrs NGOY had her period on 02 September 2022, so we're going to find the day of ovulation, the fertile days and the day of her next period:

Table 1: calculation of fertile days: normal cycle

[27] Cours de biologie, op. cit.

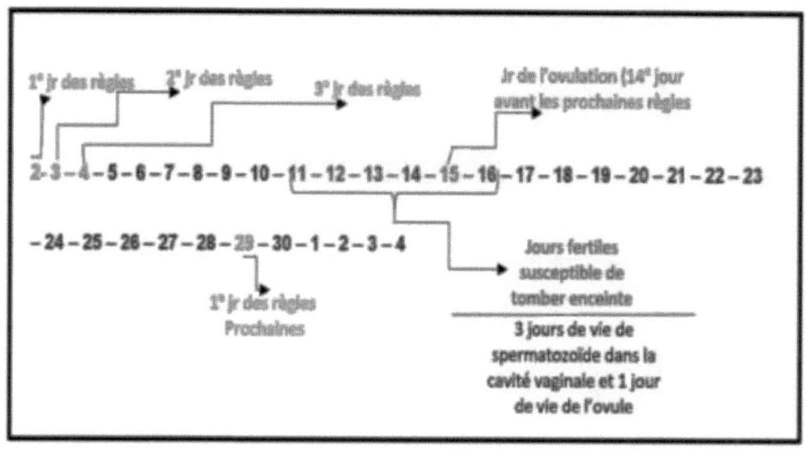

Fertilisation if you have a short cycle:

The length of the cycle varies from woman to woman. If your cycle is shorter (less than 26 days), the follicular phase is shorter and ovulation is therefore earlier. If your cycle is 21 days long, for example, ovulation takes place on the 7th^{eme} day after the first day of menstruation. The calculation is made by subtracting 14 days, the length of the luteal phase which does not vary, from the number of days in the cycle: i.e. 21 - 14 = 7. If the cycle lasts 22 days: ovulation will take place on day 8eme , i.e. 22 - 14 = 8.

Example: Mrs Ndomba has a short cycle of 21 days and her periods last 3 days. Mrs NDOMBA had her period on 02 September, so we're going to find out the day of ovulation, the fertile days and the day of her next period:

Table 2: calculation of fertile days: short cycle

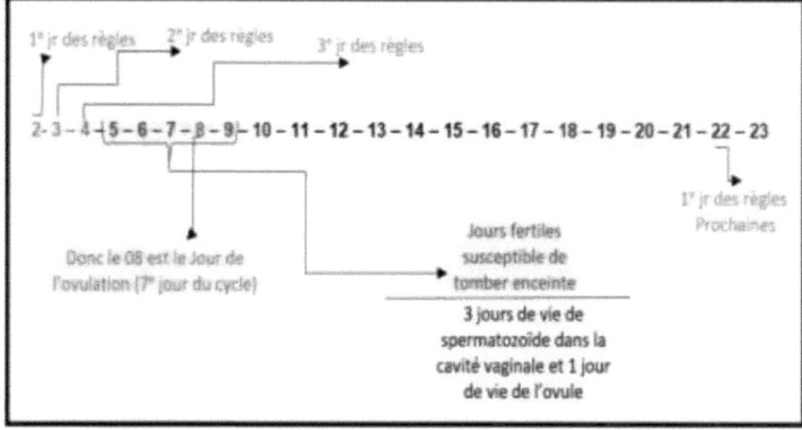

Fertilisation if you have a long cycle:

If the cycle is 33 days longer, the follicular phase is longer and ovulation occurs later (**late ovulation**), i.e. on the 19eme day from the first day of the period: i.e. 33 days - 14 days = 19 days. If the cycle lasts 34 days: ovulation takes place on day 20eme , i.e. 34 - 14 = 20.

Temperature curve

The above calculations are fairly theoretical. Making a temperature curve allows you to determine the most favourable moment to optimise your chances of getting pregnant. The diagram below shows how to draw up a temperature curve to find out exactly when you are ovulating.

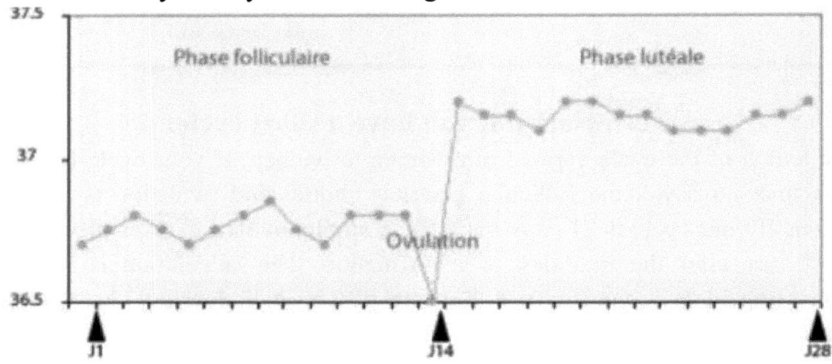

CHAPTER III

FAMILY PLANNING

What is family planning?

Family planning (FP) is the sum total of all the means and services that enable couples to have the desired number of children at the desired time, taking into account their lifestyle ethics, women's health conditions and the means available[28] .

Why family planning?

Family planning prevents abortions and maternal deaths.
Spacing births at least two years apart is one of the most important and effective strategies for reducing the number of problem births and ensuring child survival. Infants born less than two years after the birth of another child are twice as likely to die during their first year of life than infants born three years after the birth of another child. Infants and children born to mothers under the age of 20 also run a greater risk of death during the first days, months or years of their lives[29] .
In Senegal, for example, one infant in 10 born to a mother aged under 20 dies before the age of one, compared with one in 17 for women aged between 20 and 29 who have a child.
The use of family planning can prevent these deaths by enabling young women to avoid pregnancies that are too early, too unwanted and too close together. In Senegal, family planning could prevent 1.3 million unwanted pregnancies, 400,000 abortions and 200,000 deaths of children under 5 over a 10-year period.
According to a study carried out at the Katuba General Reference Hospital in the Province of Haut-Katanga in the Democratic Republic of Congo in 2020, 62.4% of the population was made up of adolescent girls aged between 14 and 19. The results of the analyses carried out show that 71.20% of the women surveyed had two living parents, compared with 28.80% of women who had no living parents. This leads us to understand that some young girls are subjected to very difficult living conditions, which leads them to adopt deviant behaviour and predisposes them to early pregnancy while still under the parental roof.
Furthermore, in the same sample, it was noted that 93.60% of women had experienced the dangers or consequences of early pregnancy, and infants born to teenage mothers were at increased risk of low birth weight, premature birth and

[28] Universite de Ouagadougou, Les methodes contraceptives, Prosad, 3e Editions July 2006.
[29] WHO, 2017

serious neonatal ailments, while 20.00% of women had pregnancies that were not carried to term for reasons that they considered confidential, but the phrase that came up most often was that "***I didn't understand how it happened***" (sic).
66.67% of women had unmarried parents compared with 33.33% of women with remarried parents; 86.00% said that the normal age for a woman to become pregnant was between 23 and 25; 100.00% of women said that they had been the victims of a bad attitude from those around them during the gestational period[30].
Family planning can prevent these deaths by enabling young women to avoid pregnancies that are too early, too unwanted and too close together.
Family planning allows couples to have the number of children they want and to choose the timing and spacing of their pregnancies, thereby improving the health of both mother and child. **Pregnancies that are too close together can be dangerous for the health of both mother and child**.
Pregnancies spaced less than 18 to 24 months apart have been associated with higher risks of premature birth, low birth weight, fatal neonatal or infant death, and adverse effects on maternal health[31].
That's why the whole point of family planning is to space out pregnancies in order to combat maternal deaths, premature births, fatal deaths, neonatal deaths, the negative effects on the mother's health, etc.
In the old days, our parents and grandparents did not expect births simply because the number of children determined the quota of supplies or bonuses received by the company (flour, milk, fish, meat, oil, tomatoes, bread, school supplies, housing, school fees, health care...).
Taking advantage of the comforts offered by the company, the only thing our parents were interested in was having a large number of children in order to benefit from the advantages granted by the most prosperous employers at the time, such as Generale des Carrieres et des Mines (GECAMINES) and Societe Nationale des Chemins de fer du Congo (SNCC), to name but two.
However, when the company closed its doors, a period of insecurity followed for heads of families, children and extended families (illness leading to death, school drop-out, severe and moderate malnutrition, loss of health, famine, increase in the illiteracy rate, increase in the number of children from broken homes, etc.). This precariousness is due to the lack of care for these children, as the Congolese state does not yet organise social security, which is limited to occasional private-sector intervention in old people's homes.
These days, the number of companies that provide this comfort to their workers

30KILANDA: la maternite precoce dans la ville de Lubumbashi, pp. 39-40, Memoire 2020.

[31] Conde-Agudelo A, Rosas-Bermudez A, Castano F, Norton MH. Effects of birth spacing on maternal, perinatal, infant, and child health: a systematic review of causal mechanisms. Studies in Family Planning, P93-114. 2012.

is hard to count; the country's economy has been at half-mast for years; reliable health infrastructures are no longer in place to provide better care in the event of complications linked to close pregnancies. And the end result is death! And the end result is death!
Based on numerous testimonies, it has been observed that many couples suffer from misinformation (intox) about family planning, leading to scenes of unwanted or undesirable births, early deaths due to poor management of repeated abortions, and an increase in the rate of children from broken families; this is followed by maternal deaths, with the consequences of the "KULUNA, CHEGUE, ATALAKU" phenomenon.
This bleak picture should encourage couples and families to engage in family planning, which is why it is so important to know how to do it, and to use appropriate methods.

When to plan

Many people would ask themselves the question of when it is possible to plan births, not knowing that they have the answer.
In the same way that a man or a woman feels the desire to get to know their partner (sexual contact), in the same way that you find yourself planning the end of year festivities according to your income, in the same way that you plan to pay for new clothes or a new telephone for your partner according to your possibilities, your financial means, a favourable circumstance and this for a given period of time.
Mutatis mutandis, you can decide **"WHEN TO DO IT"*? In other words,*** when is the right time to start family planning, taking into account your current financial situation (to educate the children, send them to school, provide them with decent medical care, cover their unmet food needs, house them, etc.) and the mother's state of health (chronic illness, incurable disease, chronic or permanent abortion or miscarriage, cesarean section, birth of triplets or twins, birth of a premature baby, emotional shock, etc.).
If you are facing some of the indicators listed above, you should sit down and think about how you can make your relationship flourish, ensure the safety of your home, protect the health of your partner, your children, your family members and the health of the people around you.

How do we get there?

As we already know, family planning (FP) is the sum total of all the means (**methods**) and services that enable couples to have the desired number of children at the desired time, taking into account the ethics of life, the health conditions of the woman and the means available.

There are several techniques or methods of contraception that can be used for successful family planning at your convenience. These methods should be chosen by mutual agreement between the partners, after a useful interview with a recognised gynaecologist, to ensure that you are protected from speculation on this subject (family planning).
This is why it is worth giving a brief outline of what needs to be done in this case when it comes to applying contraception.

Brief overview

Ensuring that all people have access to preferred methods of contraception strengthens human rights such as the right to life, the right to health, the right to maternity and the freedom to procreate, the freedom of opinion and expression, and the right to work and education, while bringing other important benefits in health and other areas.
The use of contraception protects women, particularly adolescents, from the health risks of pregnancy, and when births are less than two years apart, the infant mortality rate is 45% higher than the mortality rate when births are 2 to 3 years apart, and 60% higher than the mortality rate when births are four years or more apart.
Contraception offers a whole range of potential benefits in areas other than health, from increased opportunities for education and empowerment of women, to sustainable population growth and economic development of countries.
It should be noted, however, that the prevalence of modern methods of contraception among married women of childbearing age rose worldwide between 2000 and 2019 by 2.1 percent, from 55.0% to 57.1%[32] .
The slow rate of increase can be explained by, among other things, the limited choice of methods, limited access to services, particularly for young people, the poorest populations and unmarried people, fear or experience of side-effects, cultural or religious barriers, the poor quality of services available, biased opinions of users and providers against certain methods, and gender-related barriers to accessing services.
That said, contraceptive methods deserve to be specified.

[32] who 2017,op.cit.

CONTRACEPTIVE METHODS

Contraceptive methods are simply formulas that can be used to prevent pregnancy when you don't want to. In general, there are two types of contraceptive method:

1. natural methods of contraception ;
2. artificial contraception methods.

It's worth pointing out that neither type of contraceptive method guarantees 100% effectiveness. As you know, you can plan and decide everything, but only our supreme master, God, has the final say in all our plans and projects. "Man proposes but God disposes", they say. Psalms 127:1 "***Unless the Lord builds the house, those who build it labour in vain; Unless the Lord guards the city, those who guard it watch in vain***".

Natural contraception methods

The various natural methods include interrupted coi't, prayer, knowing your fertile days, the LAM method and abstinence, which we'll look at now.

Interrupted coitus (for men)

Interrupted coitus (*coitus interruptus* in Latin) or **the withdrawal method** is a sexual practice and a means of contraception that consists of interrupting vaginal intercourse just before ejaculation. At this point, the man withdraws his penis from the vagina and ejaculates outside it, thus avoiding fertilisation.

Prayer (for men and women)

Prayer is the communication between man and his creator (God) with the aim of satisfying our needs.

Jer. 33:3 ***"Call to me and I will answer you, and I will tell you great things, things you do not know"***.

How is prayer a method of contraception?

contraception?

One day, a couple found themselves in a precarious situation, no longer wishing to continue giving birth because they had just had twins. The woman was a servant of the Eternal Zelee; She had time to seek advice left and right on different methods of contraception, but all the methods presented to her proved to be inappropriate and she decided to invoke her God, the master of times and circumstances, the gynaecologist par excellence, to block her fertility. As if in a dream in the night, God answered his servant's prayer. Today, this couple is enjoying unprecedented fulfilment.

When you read the above testimony, you realise that prayer is indeed a method of contraception for anyone who believes in God. God knows what we need most, and it is up to us to ask him for it in accordance with his word, and with faith he will grant it to us (**I John 5:14** : We have this assurance with him that if we ask anything according to his will, he will hear us**; Psalms 37 : 5** Commit your lot to the Lord, put your trust in him, and he will act; **Philippians 4:6** Do not be anxious about anything; but in everything let your needs be made known to God by prayer and supplication, with thanksgiving).

If you don't want to use the other methods of contraception, tell God: Father, I am unable to fill the earth as you intended (GEN 1:28a God blessed them, and God said to them: ***"Be fruitful and multiply and fill the earth***"). "**In view of my financial situation, my health and the health of my children, I ask you please Father (in the name of the Lord Jesus) to stop my fertility for any length of time or for ever**.

Believe me, God is no respecter of persons. He will answer your prayer, as was the case with the couple whose testimony has just been shared. Apart from that, it's also a good idea to be familiar with the female menstrual fertility cycle.

Knowledge of fertile days (calendar, cycle necklace: woman) cycle necklace)

The fertile days, also known as the ovulatory period, are the days on which a woman is likely or probable to become pregnant. The couple avoids pregnancy by abstaining from unprotected vaginal intercourse on the most fertile days; this is calculated according to the woman's menstrual cycle (regia) using a temperature reading, calendar, etc. Please refer to the chapter on menstruation to understand the fertile days. While we're on the subject, a word about the temperature method.

The temperature method

33How[33] is this method applied ?

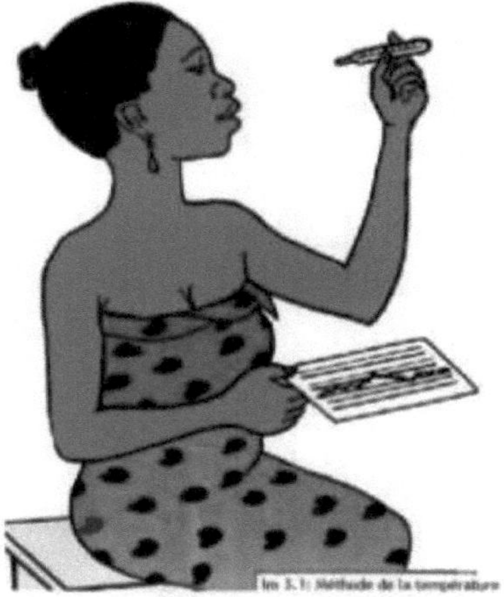

Knowing that body temperature falls by 0.5°C before ovulation and rises by 0.2 to 0.5°C at the moment of ovulation, a woman should take her temperature every morning when she wakes up at the same time and record it on a chart. She should look out for the day when the temperature rises above 37°. When this happens, she knows she is ovulating,

She remains in her fecund period until the third day after ovulation.

and therefore fecundity.

2006

With this method, women should not have sexual intercourse from the first until the third day after their temperature has risen.

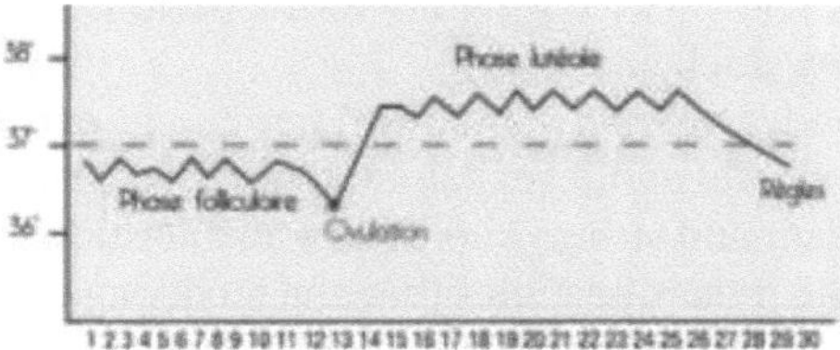

Advantages:

- It does not require medication;
- It doesn't cost much;
- Its effectiveness is good (94% to 97%);
- It is accepted by all religions;
- The woman may become pregnant as soon as the method is stopped, etc.

[33] Josephine Barry, contraceptive methods, Centre Medical Samandin, P.46-47, PROSAD

Disadvantages:

- It is not well accepted by couples because they have been abstinent for varying lengths of time,
- It does not apply to illiterate women,
- It is difficult to apply to women who work at night,
- It is difficult to apply if the woman has a fever due to illness (fever, infection...),
- It does not protect against STIs/AIDS.

Hence the need to experiment with the cervical method too.

The cervical mucus method

How is this method used?

We know that :

[34]The[34] cervical mucus is not abundant before ovulation, during
During the second period of the menstrual cycle, mucus is abundant in the

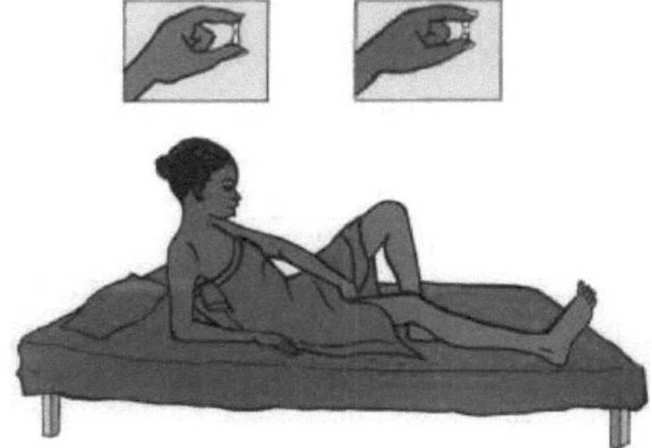

vagina. It is stringy and sticky during the fertile period. After ovulation, the mucus becomes thin, thick and sticky.

To apply this method, a woman should feel her mucus every morning when she wakes up. She should avoid sexual intercourse as soon as she notices that the mucus is abundant and stringy, i.e. sticky and elastic. She can resume intercourse when the mucus becomes thin and sticky again.

Advantages:

- It does not require medication,
- It has no financial cost,
- It gives women a better understanding of how their bodies work,
- It has no undesirable side effects on women,
- The woman can become pregnant as soon as the method is stopped.

[34] Joséphine Barry, op.cit. p;48

Disadvantages:

- She has a lot of failures,
- It requires a long apprenticeship,
- It requires a period of abstinence of varying lengths,
- It does not protect against STIs/AIDS,
- There is a risk of infection.

This suggests the idea of also using the method of sexual abstinence.

Abstinence (for women and men)

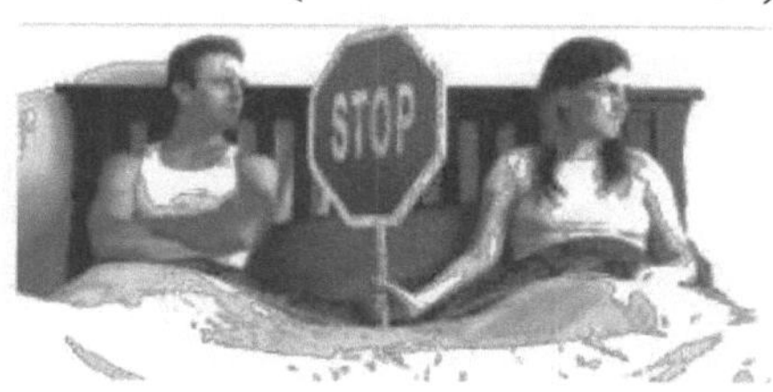

This method is particularly recommended for young single people. If you are old enough to get married, get married. If not, use
of total abstinence to combat the social damage described above.

Advantages:

- There is no possibility of pregnancy,
- It does not require medication, - It is not expensive.

Disadvantages:

- It's hard to bear,
- It exposes both partners to sexual vagrancy,
- It can cause misunderstandings in the home.

In doing so, gynaecologists sometimes suggest something else:

The fixed day method (MJF) (CYCLE COLLAR)

The Fixed Day Method (FDM), known as the Cycle Collar, is a natural method based on knowledge of the menstrual cycle.

Description of the cycle collar :

It's a necklace made up of different coloured beads representing each day of a woman's menstrual cycle. It can help a woman to know when she might become pregnant following unprotected sex.

- The white beads mark the days when you can get pregnant,
- Maroon beads mark the days when you're unlikely to get pregnant,
- A black cylinder with an arrow indicating which way to move the ring.

Who can use the cycle collar

- Women who want a natural, effective method of family planning,
- Women with cycles between 26 and 32 days.

How to use the cycle collar

- On the first day of your period, place the ring on the red bead, 35- Mark[35] the first day of your period on your calendar. You need to know this day in case you forget to move the ring,

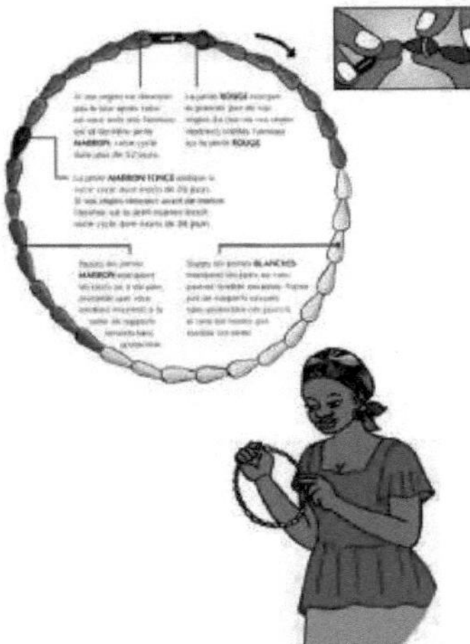

- Every morning, move the ring in the direction of the arrow on the cylinder,
- Keep moving the ring every day, from bead to bead, even on days when you have your period,
- The day your next period comes, put the ring back on the RED bead. If you have any brown beads left, skip them,
- When the ring is on a WHITE bead, you can become pregnant through unprotected sex,
- When the ring is on a BROWN bead, it is unlikely that you will become pregnant as a result of unprotected sex.

Advantages

- It's a natural method and has no side effects,
- No medication or surgery is required,
- Simple method, easy to teach, easy to use,
- A 95% effective method (when used correctly), it considerably reduces the likelihood of an unwanted pregnancy,
- Very low-cost method,
- Involves both partners by offering opportunities to improve communication within the couple.

Its disadvantages

- Does not protect against STI/HIV/AIDS,

[35] Josephine Barry, Op.cit. p;49

- it requires sexual abstinence on fertile days or the use of an effective barrier method.

In addition, the MAMA method should be tried out

MAMA (for women)

The LAM method is based on breastfeeding and amenorrhea.

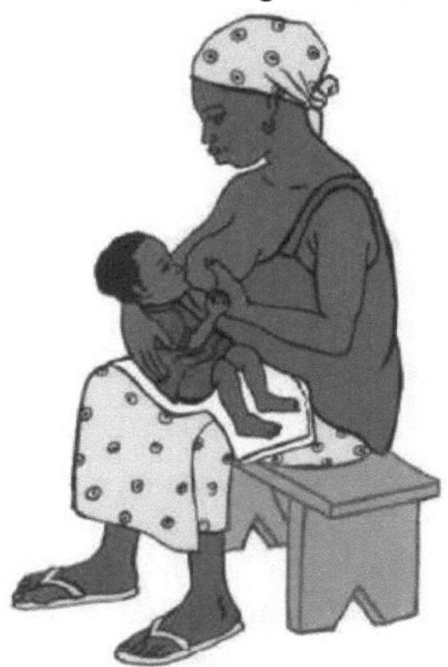

Prolactin, a hormone released in sufficient quantities in the body of a woman who is fully breastfeeding, considerably reduces the release[36] of the hormones required for ovulation to resume. The LAM method provides the mother with effective contraception for up to 6 months after childbirth if she is fully breastfeeding and all the following conditions are met:

- breastfeeding on demand: day and night with a minimum of 6 teats per 24 hours and never more than 6 hours between teats;
- Exclusive breastfeeding: the baby receives no solids or liquids other than milk taken directly from the breast and does not use a pacifier;
- absence of menstruation; less than 6 months have elapsed since the birth.

Efficiency

98% efficiency if all conditions are met.

Advantages:

- it's not expensive;
- it encourages breast-feeding;
- it does not require medication;
- it is accepted by all religions;

[3636] Josephine Barry, Op.cit, Pp.50

- a woman can become pregnant as soon as she stops using this method;
- no side effects, etc.

Disadvantages:

- 1 breastfeeding on demand, including at night, is difficult for mothers to bear;
- the method is only valid for 6 months;
- exclusive breastfeeding is not yet universally accepted;
- ovulation may occur without the mother's knowledge and she may well become pregnant;
- it does not protect against STIs/AIDS;
- is not recommended for women with debilitating illnesses (HIV/AIDS, tuberculosis, cancer, severe heart disease).

In addition to the natural methods described, the following artificial contraception methods should also be considered:

Artificial contraception

These methods have different modes of action and are effective in preventing unwanted pregnancy.

It should be noted that before making the right choice from among these methods, the man and/or woman should be given full explanations and details (advantages and disadvantages) relating to each method. And this information can only come from a qualified gynaecologist.

To choose a contraceptive method that **suits you and your lifestyle**, it is important to consider the following points:

- your schedule and lifestyle;
- the effectiveness of the method ;
- the advantages and disadvantages associated with this method;
- contraindications and your state of health.

The various artificial contraceptive methods include :

- The implant
- The contraceptive pill
- The patch
- The vaginal ring
- Cervical cap
- The diaphragm
- The female condom
- The hormonal IUD and the copper IUD
- Sterilisation
- Spermicides

- Injectable contraceptives
- Emergency contraception

1. The implant

[37]The implant is the size of a match and is inserted at the level of the on the inside of the arm, under the skin, and diffuses a hormone that blocks

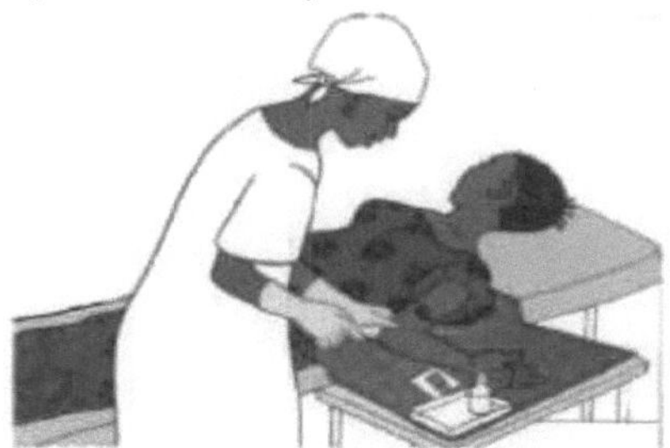

ovulation. This method of contraception is effective for 3 years and 99.9% reliable, but does not protect against sexually transmitted diseases. The doctor or midwife inserts the implant under local anaesthetic, which only lasts a few minutes. It can be removed as soon as you wish, but cannot remain in place for more than 3 years.

The benefits of contraceptive implants

- Simple and long-lasting: after installation, you're protected for 3 years.
- Discretion and comfort: inserted under the skin of the arm, 1 implant goes unnoticed.
- Installation and removal are quick and easy.

The disadvantages of the contraceptive implant

The contraceptive implant may cause side effects such as :

- **Changes in menstrual cycles**: some women will not have periods for 3 years. Others will have **periods** that are **less regular** or **less frequent** than usual; sometimes much shorter, sometimes longer. If you are bothered or tired by this irregular bleeding, don't hesitate to talk to your doctor.
- **Weight gain for some women** (if you weigh more than 80 kilos, it is advisable to change the implant earlier (after 24 to 30 months, not 3 years).
- **Acne in some women** (pimples on the face).

2. The contraceptive pill

[38]While the contraceptive pill is 99.7% reliable in theory, it does not

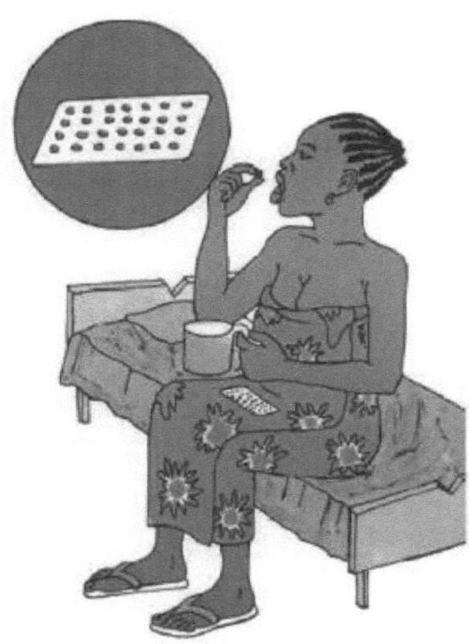

1 is only 91% effective in practice (forgetfulness, interaction with other medicines, etc.). The pill must be taken at the same time every day for 21 days followed by a 7-day break, or 28 days depending on the pill, and does not protect against 1STS.

The benefits of the contraceptive pill

- Menstruation is less abundant, more regular, lasts less time and is often less painful.
- The pill can reduce acne.
- You can stop taking anything

without consulting a doctor, and the return to fertility is easy.
fast.

- The pill is readily available from chemists.

The disadvantages of the contraceptive pill

- It should be taken every day, at roughly the same time.
- You need a medical prescription to obtain them.

[38] Henry Joyeux, contraceptive pill Pp.163-168, Editions du Rocher, 2013

The benefits

- It doesn't cost much;
- It is very effective;
- It is available in health centres and pharmacies;
- A woman can become pregnant again within a reasonable time after stopping the pill;
- It relieves certain illnesses;
- It regularises irregular cycles;

- It does not cause genital infections in women;
- It is independent of sexual activity;
- It can be provided by trained non-medical staff.

Side effects:

- Vaginal bleeding ;
- Breast tension ;
- Headaches;
- No rules ;
- Nausees ;
- Vomiting, dizziness, acnes ;
- Weight gain ;
- Reduced milk secretion in women who breastfeed;
- Chest pain;
- Elevation of blood pressure ;
- Reduced sexual pleasure.

Its disadvantages

- It requires medical supervision;
- It is difficult to take;
- It has many contraindications;
- It reduces milk production in breastfeeding women;
- It does not protect against STI/HIV/AIDS.

Health risks and contraindications of the contraceptive pill

Although widely used, the contraceptive pill presents a number of **health risks**, including the risk of blood clots, strokes and high blood pressure. There are also **contraindications to** taking the pill. For example, if :

- you're over 35; you smoke or have migraines;
- you get migraines with aura (fever);
- you are breastfeeding ;
- you have a history of blood clots, stroke or heart problems.

3. The patch

[39]Like the pill, the patch is an effective method of contraception (99.7% in theory, 91% in practice). It is placed on the skin (away from the breasts) and releases hormones to block ovulation. The patch must

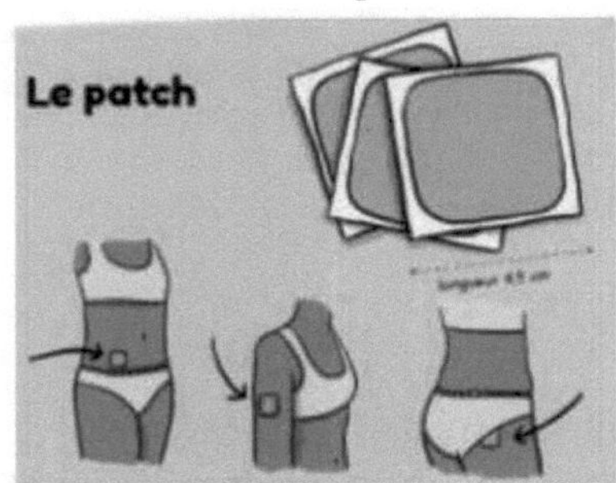

to be repeated every week, 3 times a month at the same time.

If the patch is not applied during the last week, this does not mean that you are not protected: the contraceptive effect is still present. Stopping the patch simply causes your period to start.

The benefits

- **Duration of action**: the patch is active for one week, reducing the risk of forgetting to take the pill.
- **Easy to use**: it sticks to the skin, so you can check that it's in place.

Disadvantages and contraindications

- **Possible side effects**: nausea, painful swelling of the breasts, bleeding, headaches...
- **Visible** to the partner or if the woman is in a swimming costume.
- **Risk of detachment** (rate of detachment is less than 2% - 1.8% total detachment and 2.9% partial detachment) but it is possible to refasten it or fit another within 24 hours.

Note that women for whom **the combined pill is contraindicated** cannot use the contraceptive patch.

4. The vaginal ring

[40]The vaginal ring delivers hormones continuously. It

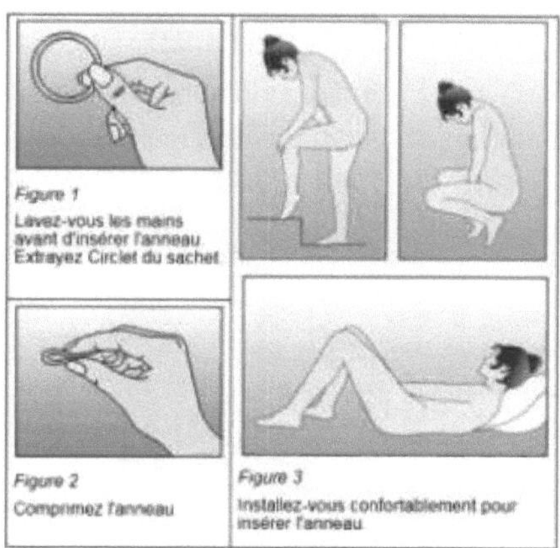

is approximately 5 cm in diameter. It is flexible and is placed in the vagina in the same way as a tampon. It is left in place for 3 weeks, and removed in the fourth week, always at the same time. This triggers your period. You should be aware that even if you have removed your ring, you are still protected against an unwanted pregnancy during the 7-day break. It does not protect against STIs.

When used perfectly, the contraceptive ring is as effective as a pill or patch: it provides 99.7% protection. The risk of forgetting to take it is reduced, as you only have to think about it every 3 weeks.

Benefits

It allows you to benefit from **effective contraception without having to think about it for 3 weeks**. This makes the vaginal ring a suitable method for women who tend to forget their pill. It's worth remembering that a quarter of all abortions are due to accidents involving the pill.

Another advantage: the contraceptive ring delivers hormones at a lower dose and on a more regular basis than oral contraception.

Inconveniences and contraindications

The contraindications are broadly the same as those for the pill: history of venous or arterial thrombosis, diabetes, severe liver disease, suspected hormone-dependent tumours. This is why its use should be discussed with your gynaecologist.

This device is also not recommended for women suffering from uterine prolapse or constipation, **due to** an increased risk of accidental expulsion. In this case, the ring can be rinsed out with warm water and replaced, while retaining its effectiveness. However, this incident, as well as **sensations of a foreign body** or **discomfort during sexual intercourse**, are extremely limited. Uterine prolapse means the displacement of the uterus in its proper place.

5. The diaphragm and cervical cap

The diaphragm is a cup of variable size or size which is placed at the bottom of the vagina to block the passage of urine.

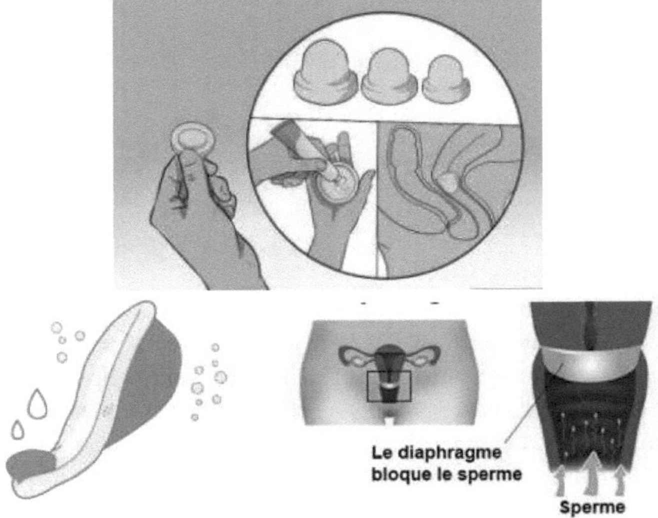

spermatozoa worms

the uterus. It is made of silicone. It is used in combination with a spermicide (a product that destroys spermatozoa) to increase its effectiveness.

The cap is a very thin silicone dome that covers the cervix.

41The diaphragm or cervical cap can be fitted at the time of intercourse, or several hours before. It is important to keep them in place for 8 hours after intercourse. They can be reused.

The Diaphragm is 94% effective when used correctly. The **cervical** cap is 91% effective in women who have not had children, and 74% effective in women who have already been pregnant.

The advantages of the diaphragm

- The contraceptive effect of the diaphragm is prolonged, regardless of the number of sexual encounters.
- It does not interfere with the hormonal system, cycle length or blood flow.
- It can be used during breastfeeding.
- It can only be used when necessary.

The disadvantages of the diaphragm

- There may be difficulties with insertion and removal.
- The diaphragm must be prescribed by a doctor, who will carry out an examination to measure the cervix.

- The diaphragm can cause urinary or vaginal infections.

Health risks and contraindications of the contraceptive patch

The diaphragm is contraindicated if :

- You have a lot of urinary or vaginal infections
- You have a cervical anomaly
- You have an allergy to silicone, latex or spermicide.

6. The female/male condom

The female condom blocks spermatozoids and protects against 1ST. It is an effective form of protection (95% in theory, 79% in practice) that prevents fertilisation without the need for hormones.

The male condom is highly reliable when used correctly (98%), it also protects against 1ST and does not require any hormonal treatment. The male condom is for single use only and is placed on the erect penis during each sexual encounter.

A. Male condom or condom: the problem of spacing and numbering !!!!!!

[42]It's[47] a thin envelope made of rubber or a natural product.

which is placed on the penis during erection before sexual intercourse to

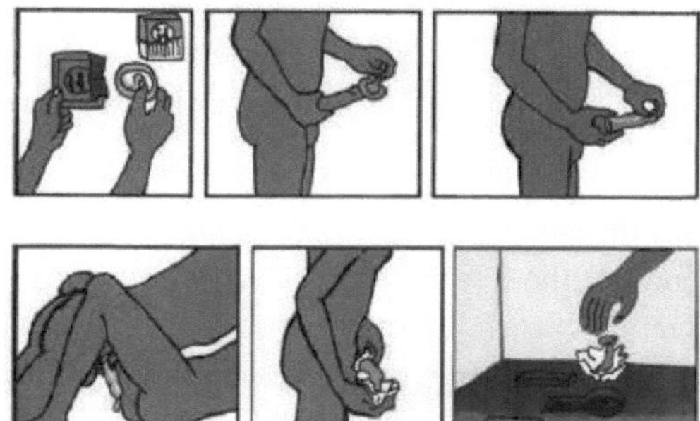

prevent sperm from coming into contact with the woman's genital tract.

How do condoms help prevent pregnancy?

The condom prevents sperm from entering the woman's vagina.

Advantages:

- It doesn't cost much;
- It is available everywhere on the market;
- It has few side effects;
- It protects against 1ST and HIV/AIDS;

[47][42] Josephine Barry, Op.cit, Pp.52

- It is suitable for occasional sex;
- It protects against unwanted pregnancies;
- She doesn't need a prescription;
- It involves men in family planning;
- It works immediately;
- It does not affect breastfeeding;
- Can be used in addition to other methods.

Disadvantages:

- The condom reduces the sensitivity of the glans;
- Some men cannot maintain erection to wear a condom;
- The preliminaries have to be interrupted before the condom can be worn;
- use a single condom each time you have sex;
- Effectiveness depends on willingness to follow advice.

Side effects:

Some people are allergic to latex

How is the condom used?

- Before intercourse :

- Wash your hands with soap and water (if possible),
- Wait until the penis is erect,
- check that the packaging is correct,
- check the expiry date,
- Mark the saw-tooth edge of the packaging,
- Carefully tear off the packaging at the saw teeth,
- Remove the bonnet without tearing it,
- Identify the direction of travel,
- Pinch the tapered end between your thumb and forefinger to expel the air,
- Place the cap over the top of the glans, holding the tip between your fingers,
- Untie the condom over the penis to the root,
- Begin intercourse by gently penetrating your partner.

- After intercourse

- Remove the penis from the vagina before the end of erection, holding the condom against the penis with your fingers to prevent it from remaining in the vagina or sperm from escaping,
- Once the penis has been removed, remove the condom and dispose of it safely. If the partners wish to have sex again, the man must wear another condom,
- Wash your hands after removing the condom.

Oй do you find condoms?

The condom is available from a number of outlets: aprons, health centres, pharmacies and community workers. They can be purchased without a prescription.

B. The female condom

The female condom is a barrier method to protect against STI/HIV/AIDS and unwanted pregnancies.

Characteristics of the female condom :

Shape: like a bag closed at the end with two rings,

A ring with a floating interior that allows the female condom to be inserted easily into the vagina and held in place at the bottom of the vagina, and **another** with a fixed end that serves to hold it in place by covering the external parts of the sex.

Dimensions: 17 cm deep; 7.8 cm diameter; 0.42-0.53 mm thick.

Material: polyurethane (male condoms are made of latex or vinyl), transparent, flexible, lubricated, odourless, single-use.

The benefits

- Immediately effective,
- Strong and resistant (does not tear easily),
- No allergies,
- Women are autonomous and responsible for their sexuality,
- Fits all sizes of vagina,
- Covers the entire vagina and vulva of the woman herself,
- Can be worn 8 hours before intercourse,
- No interruption of sexual activity like the male condom (can be inserted 8 hours before intercourse),
- Easy to use after several tries,
- Allows partners to stay a little longer in each other's arms after sex,
- No prescription required,
- Protects against STIs/AIDS and unwanted pregnancies,
- Does not affect breast-feeding,
- Can be controlled by the woman.

Its disadvantages

- High cost compared with male condoms,
- Difficult to insert when first used,
- [48]Reduced sexual position. Only the missionary position allows comfortable. This is a position in which the woman lies on her back with her legs spread, while the man penetrates her between her legs,
- Can only be used once during each sexual encounter,

[48] Josephine Barry, Op.cit, Pp.53

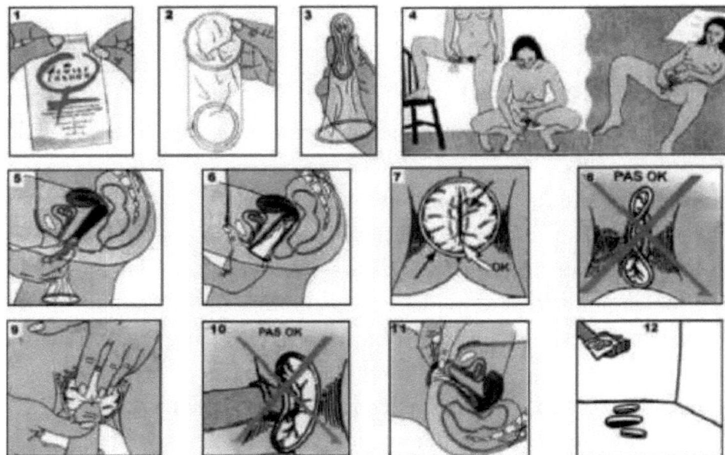

- Effectiveness depends on willingness to follow instructions.

How to use the female condom

- Wash hands with soap,
- Knead the packaging to distribute the lubricant evenly,
- Open the packaging with your fingers, following the arrow, without using sharp objects,
- Pinch the inner ring between the index finger and thumb or with the middle finger in the shape of an 8,
- Choose a suitable position (squat or rest your leg on a chair or stool, or lie on your back with your legs slightly bent).
- Spread the large lips of the vulva with the other hand and introduce the female condom in the vagina,
- [49] Using one or two fingers inside the female condom push the ring as far as possible to ensure that it is firmly fixed at the bottom of the vagina, around the cervix, and does not twist,
- The outer ring remains outside the vagina and covers the external parts of the sex,
- During penetration, hold the ring and help the man by putting his sex in the middle of the female condom to prevent the penis from slipping past,
- To remove the female condom after ejaculation, use a tissue or toilet paper to hold the outer ring, rotate it and remove it before standing up,
- Wrap it up, put it in the bin or bury it and wash your hands,

The female condom is used only once.

[49] Henry Joyeux, Op.cit. Pp.170-175.

Ой where can I find the female condom?

- In health facilities,
- In pharmacies,
- Community agents, certain associations.

7. The hormonal IUD and the copper IUD

The IUD (or Intra Uterine Device), better known as a "***sterilet***", is a reliable means of contraception (over 99%) placed in the uterus by a health professional every 4 to 10 years. However, it can be removed by the doctor as soon as the woman wishes.

The hormonal IUD regularly releases a progestin hormone which thickens the secretions from the cervix of[50] the uterus and blocks the passage of spermatozoa. It also reduces the volume and duration of menstrual periods.

The copper IUD works without hormones, as the copper renders the sperm inactive. On the other hand, it has no effect on the length or volume of menstrual periods.

The advantages and disadvantages

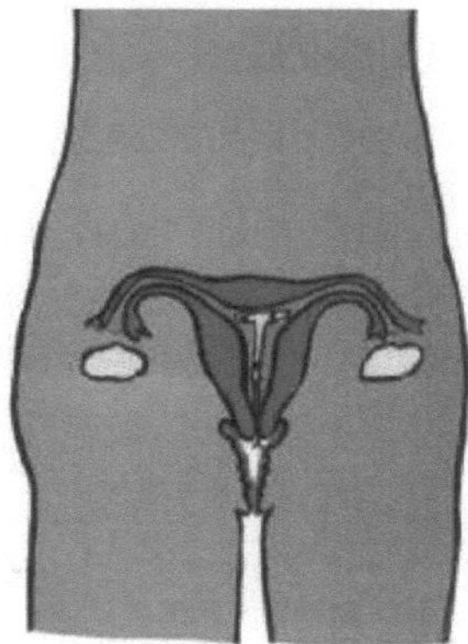

- Simple and long-lasting: after application, you are protected for 4 to 10 days, depending on the model.

• Comfort: you won't feel the device and it won't affect your partner during sex.

• No hormones: copper renders sperm inactive.

On the other hand, the Copper can make your periods last longer. But if your periods are short and light, the difference will be imperceptible.

Copper IUD: contraindications

Not eligible for a copper IUD:

[50] Ditto

- Women with a **malformation of the uterus** or a large fibroid and those whose **cervix is too large** (due to multiple or difficult deliveries).
- Women with **cervical or endometrial cancer** (before treatment).
- Women **who have had a 1ST** less than 3 months ago.
- Women with **an upper genital infection** (of the uterus or fallopian tubes) that is ongoing, recurrent or less than 3 months old.
- Women with **unexplained vaginal bleeding.**
- Women who **have just given birth** (you need to wait between 48 hours and 4 weeks after giving birth).
- Women who have had **an infection following childbirth or an abortion less than 3 months ago**.
- Women who **have** had **genital tuberculosis**.

Note that you can have a sterilet inserted even if you have not had children (if there are no contraindications). The copper IUD comes in two sizes, "short" and "standard". So there's one to suit every size of uterus.

Contraindications of the hormonal IUD

Contrary to popular belief, the hormonal IUD **is not reserved for women who have already had children**. It also has the advantage of being highly effective, having a long duration of action and posing no risk of cancer or cardiovascular disease.

However, there are a number of contraindications to its use:

- Previous uterine or trophoblastic pathologies (including certain anomalies),
- Recent or ongoing vaginal pathologies, unexplained vaginal/genital bleeding,
- Various infectious risk situations (STDs, hepatitis genital infections, etc.)
- Hypersensitivity to one of the ingredients,
- Immediate post-partum (between 48 hours and 4 weeks)
- Suspected or known pregnancy.

For levonorgestrel hormonal IUDs, the few **contraindications inherent in the use of a progestin should also be taken into account** (deep vein thrombosis, current pulmonary embolism, migraine with neurological symptoms, current breast cancer or breast cancer in remission for less than 5 years, liver disease, current ischaemic heart disease).

The advantages and disadvantages

- Simple and long-lasting: after application, you are protected for 4 to 10 days, depending on the model.
- Comfort: you won't feel the device and it won't affect your partner during sex.

- Effects on **painful and heavy areas**

On the other hand, the hormonal IUD can cause the same side effects as contraceptives containing progestins.

8. Female and male sterilisation

Female sterilisation is generally definitive and can be achieved by tubal ligation or hysteroscopy.

Male sterilisation, better known as a vasectomy, is a definitive operation that consists of blocking or severing the ducts that allow sperm to pass from the testicles to the penis. This surgical procedure is performed by a urologist or uro-andrologist and lasts just a few minutes. After the operation, the man can still have an erection and ejaculate, but his sperm is now sperm-free. Male sterilisation is a 99.8% effective contraceptive.

Tubal ligation: risks and complications

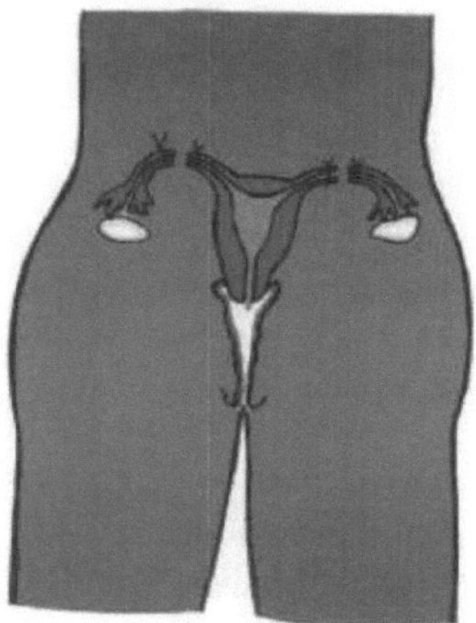

46 Post-operative complications are rare and generally benign. Most often, they consist of abdominal pain or small abdominal pains.
temporary bleeding.

Like all surgical operations, a risk of infection cannot be ruled out (although this is rare). And in less than 1% of cases, tubal ligation fails. In the latter case, the woman is at increased risk of an ectopic pregnancy. Any delay in menstruation should therefore be reported to a doctor.

Vasectomy: what are the side effects?

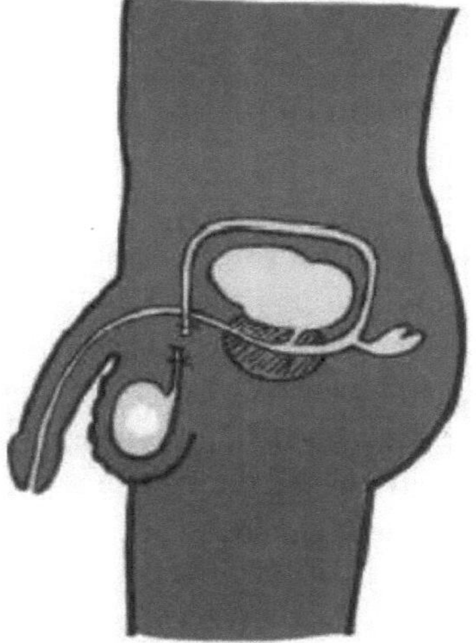

[47]The efficacy[51] of vasectomy is very high. However, in a very small percentage of patients (between 1 and 3%), spontaneous recanalisation of the vas deferens may occur. In order to be sure of the success of vasectomy, patients are invited to have different post-operative spermograms after a certain period of time. If the analysis of the ejaculate concludes that there are no spermatozoa **(azoospermia)**, sterilisation will be confirmed.

Some men may also develop immune reactions to spermatozoids. In other words, they develop antibodies against sperm.

48But its main disadvantage is paradoxically linked to its effectiveness. As we have already emphasised, this operation must be considered as definitive sterilisation. Extreme care must therefore be taken with pre-operative advice.

9. Spermicides

Spermicides are substances that destroy or render inactive spermatozoids. The use of spermicides is an emergency contraceptive method that is not very effective. Spermicides are

[5147] Josephine Barry, op.cit. p; 62

[48] Ditto

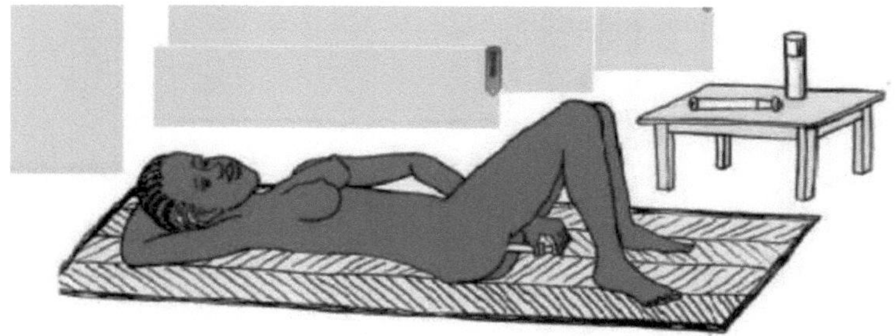

come in gel or ovule form. They are placed in the vagina before each act of intercourse. It is advisable to use them in conjunction with another method of contraception, such as a diaphragm or cervical cap. Spermicides can also be combined with male condoms to lubricate the vaginal wall and increase their effectiveness.

The effectiveness of spermicides is highly variable, as it is not always known exactly when penetration will take place. Cream spermicides must be inserted before intercourse and last for around 8 hours. Ova take 10 minutes to melt and work for 60 minutes. Given these constraints, the failure rate varies between 18 and 29%.

Their advantages:

- They're easy to buy,
- They're very easy to use,
- They are ideal for occasional sex,
- They are affordable.

Their disadvantages:

- There are a lot of failures,
- They can cause lesions on the penis or in the vagina,
- You should wait ten (10) minutes before having sexual intercourse,
- Their presence in the vagina affects sexual intercourse (burning, tingling, rubbing, inflammation of the vagina...),
- They do not protect against STIs/AIDS.

10. Injectable contraceptives

An injectable contraceptive, i.e. a hormone, is administered by intramuscular injection every 3 months by a doctor, nurse or midwife. This ensures continuous contraception for 12 weeks. This method is very effective, but it can cause significant undesirable effects (weight gain, delayed menstruation, etc.) that cannot be prevented, only by waiting for the effects to cease.

Like the pill or patch, injectable progestins are more than 99.7% effective when

used perfectly. Omissions and errors

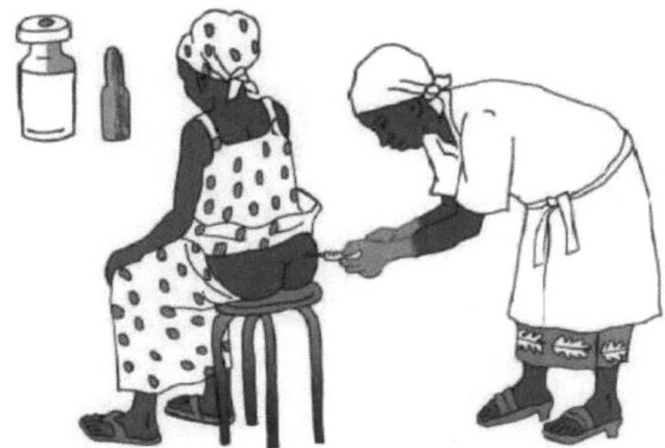

use reduces its average effectiveness to 4991%. There is a risk that its effects may be diminished by the use of drugs that inhibit hormones (drugs used to treat epilepsy, tuberculosis, depression, etc.). This risk therefore also applies to all other hormonal contraceptive methods.

The benefits of contraceptive injections

- This method does not require daily attention.
- The injection can be used by people who are unable to take restrogens.
- The injection may be administered during breast-feeding.

The disadvantages of contraceptive injections

- The biggest drawback of the contraceptive injection is that if you want to stop taking it, for example if you're too bothered by the side effects, you have to wait until it has worn off, i.e. three months after the injection.
- Injections require a medical prescription and appointments are made every three months.
- The return to fertility may take longer than with other methods of contraception.

11. Emergency contraception

[50]If you forget to take the pill, or if the condom breaks during intercourse, emergency contraception (or the morning-after pill) can help prevent an unwanted pregnancy.

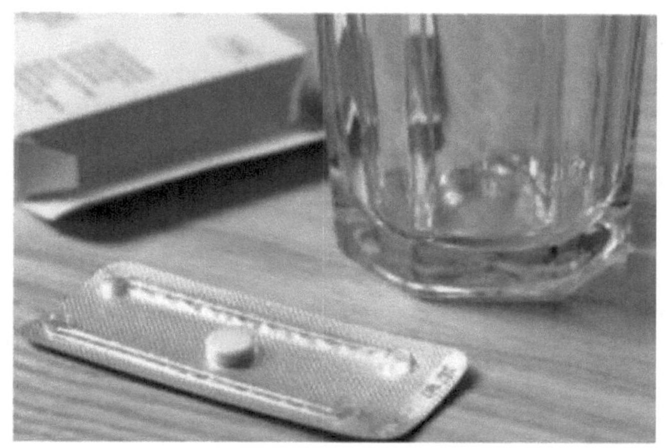

CONCLUSION

Having skimmed through this book, I can't wait to read it and savour its content, which sheds more light on the lanterns that light up people's imaginations when it comes to questions about virginity, menstruation and family planning.

Virginity is a question that many people take in a context that is not particularly their own or appropriate. But as we read through this book, we were all made aware of our own grey areas. Virginity, a word used by many in the limelight, and many couples, families and young girls have fallen victim to it, having suffered atrocities because of the misconception of this word; divorces have followed after the wedding, leaving the married woman to her sad fate, with numerous consequences: abandonment of children by their parents, abandonment of the bride by her husband, and all these consequences lead to a depravation of morals. Thanks to this book, we will have fewer consequences linked to the misconception of the term "***virginity***".

Menstruation is another important issue, but one that is often neglected by the needy and less often presented to beneficiaries by healthcare staff. This reality leads to unfortunate consequences in the community: early and unwanted pregnancies, abortions, etc., all of which lead to maternal death.This book will help us to clear up the ambiguity surrounding the calculation of fertile and non-fertile days, and to avoid panicking about irregular periods, menstrual cycle dysfunction and the colour and smell of menstrual periods, so that we don't fall victim to the evils that lie at the root of misinformation on this subject.

When it comes to family planning, two words can come out of your union: "***a Choice***" and a "***Decision***" to fight against the depravation of the masses due to the lack of accurate and coherent information to decide when, how and why births are desirable.

Remember that God gave man and woman fertility in order to fulfil his will to multiply, but it is up to man and woman to manage this fertility rationally.

Poor management of childbearing gives rise to the ATALAKU, SHEGUE (children from broken families) phenomenon, and these children are a source of concern for the population in terms of safety, premature death, maternal death, disorientation in life, overcrowding (global warming), pollution beyond the norm, abortions... with all their consequences, even though the Maputo Protocol authorises medical abortion but under limited conditions.

This is the place to look ahead to 2030. What will living conditions be like on this planet? Parents, couples, carers, political and health authorities, let's all get out of the way of irrational fertility management.

REFERENCES BIBLIOGRAPHIQUES

LEGAL INSTRUMENTS AND RESOURCES

- Protocol to the African Charter on Human and Peoples' Rights on the Rights of Women in Africa.
- Constitution of the Democratic Republic of Congo
- Law N° 06/015 of 12 June 2006 authorising the Democratic Republic of Congo to accede to the Protocol to the African Charter on Human and Peoples' Rights on the Rights of Women in Africa
- Congolese penal code.
- Family Code

BOOKS

- Henry JOYEUX, ***Pilule contraceptive***, P.163-200, Editions du Rocher, 2013 Yvonne KNIBIEHLER, ***La Virginite feminine: Mythes, fantasmes, emancipation,*** 2012.

MAGAZINES AND NEWSPAPERS

- Journal des femmes, Paris.
- Journal Le Monde, 24 September 2017 and 7 May 2022.
- Pauline MORTAS, Une Rose epineuse. La defloration au XIXe siecle en France, Rennes, Presses Universitaires de Rennes, coll, 2017.
- Danielle BOUGAIRE: contraceptive methods. University of Ouagadougou 2006.
- Josephine BARRY/WAONGO: Centre Medical Samandin: les methodes contraceptives. University of Ouagadougou 2006
- Trong HIEU DINH, "Vraies et fausses vierges au Viet Nam. La falsification corporelle en question", Extreme-Orient Extreme- Occident, no 32, 1er October2010 , p. 163-191 (ISSN 0754 5010, DOI 10.4000/extremeorient.115, read online [archive], consulted on 7 January 2020).
- Fil sante jeunes "Virginity, what is it? [archive], (consulted on 7 January 2020).
- World Health Organization: prevalence and risk of early pregnancy, 2017
- Conseil national de l'ordre des sages-femmes: Annex to the practical information sheet on contraception - COVID19: Tools for teleconsultation on contraception and sexual health (Paris 2020).

DICTIONARIES

- Dictionary of the French Academy

COURSES

- Biology course, 6e des humanites Scientifiques, Complexe Scolaire des Eloges, 2012.

WEB SITES

- www.choisirsacontraception.fr (consulted on 15 September 2021).
- www.onsexprime.fr/ www.info-ist.fr(consulted on 15 September 2021).

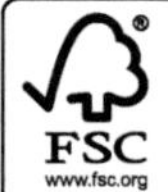

MIX
Papier aus verantwortungsvollen Quellen
Paper from responsible sources
FSC® C105338

Printed by Books on Demand GmbH, Norderstedt / Germany